12 Essential Minerals
for Cellular Health

12 Essential Minerals for Cellular Health

An Introduction to Cell Salts

David R. Card

KALINDI PRESS
Chino Valley, Arizona

Cover design: Zachary Parker
Layout and design: Zachary Parker, Kadak Graphics

ISBN: 978-1-935826-39-2

KALINDI PRESS
P.O. Box 4410
Chino Valley, AZ 86323
800-381-2700
www.kalindipress.com

CONTENTS

Contents

PREFACE

As a homeopathic practitioner, I have used cell salts for several years with gratifying results. Recently, I completed a six-month practical study on the effects of cell salts in sixty-three people. Although personal results varied, you will read their positive comments throughout this book.

Cell salts have always been considered an important part of healing in homeopathy. They have been neglected in the English-speaking part of the world for many years. In this book I am bringing them back to light, where you will find easy, applicable ways to use them. The cell salts are available in most healthfood stores, and their healing power is available to every family. You can also find cell salts at www.daveshealth.com.

Much of what has been written on cell salts is in older medical language, which may be hard to understand. Here, cell salts are explained in a more comprehensive fashion, simply, and in our modern language. You will also find a section on external uses, something seldom revealed in the English language.

Anyone can use this system to find fast and lasting health benefits. Every family needs cell salts to improve their health and prevent possible illness. Share this book with your friends or family, and have better health.

– David R. Card

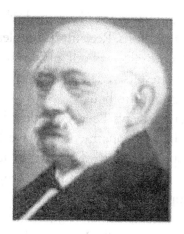

Dr. Wilhelm Schuessler

CHAPTER 1
An Introduction to Cell Salts

Dr. Wilhelm Schuessler, a medical doctor born in Germany in the 1800s, incorporated homeopathy into his practice with great success. He also learned from the early pioneers of biochemistry about **12 Essential Minerals** required for cellular health, namely:

- Calc Fluor (calcium fluoride)
- Calc Phos (calcium phosphate)
- Calc Sulph (calcium sulphate)
- Ferrum Phos (iron)
- Kali Mur (potassium chloride)
- Kali Phos (potassium phosphate)
- Kali Sulph (potassium sulphate)
- Mag Phos (magnesium phosphate)
- Nat Mur (sodium chloride)
- Nat Phos (sodium phosphate)
- Nat Sulph (sodium sulphate)
- Silicea (silica)

Healthy cells amount to a healthy person. Dr. Schuessler found that the lack of one or more of these 12 minerals (often called **tissue salts**) put the body out of balance and into "dis-ease." He developed them homeopathically, so they could be easily taken and assimilated. Many of the conditions that we experience today are due to the lack of particular minerals in our bodies.

Schuessler cell salts are the 12 minerals essential to the body's functions. In their preparation, these minerals are ground finely into milk sugar and diluted, so they become small enough to be absorbed by the tissues of the body, internally or externally. In this form they can go right to the cells of our tissues.

These tissue salts provide harmonious cellular chemistry for optimal health, which is why they are more commonly known as **cell salts**. When our cells are deficient in minerals, we experience loss of energy, unclear thinking, or emotional discomfort. This is where cell salts shine. They quickly get minerals to our cells to help us regain or maintain our health.

All bodily functions and conditions are influenced on a cellular level by these essential minerals; therefore **they can help any condition or disease. The signs of deficiency of these minerals can be seen by looking at a person's face.** The technique of facial diagnosis has been used for years. Signs of deficiency can be seen in the texture or color of skin, puffiness, dryness, lines, etc.

As a nutritionist, herbalist, and homeopathic practitioner, I have found that cell salts tend to be overlooked in Homeopathy. After reading a German book about how to read mineral deficiencies on a person's face (*Antlitzdiagnostik* by Peter Emmrich), I began to use cell salts and study facial diagnosis of mineral deficiencies in my own practice. The results were astonishing! People began asking for more information, so I wrote the book *Facial Diagnosis of Cell Salt Deficiencies* (Hohm Press, 2005). I also had an artist draw what the deficiencies look like for each of the twelve tissue remedies. These drawings were included in "The Power of Cell Salts Seminar" which I presented in Salt Lake City, Utah in October of 2005. That month we began a practical study with our customers, done over a six-month period with sixty-three cases. You will see comments from study participants throughout this book.

Cell salts may be taken internally, or used externally in creams, baths, or sprays. Cell salts are generally used in the 6x potency (strength). There are several manufacturers, but I prefer the Hyland's brand because it is easily accessible at most health-food stores. There are also many other fine brands.

Cell salts in lactose are soft and dissolve within seconds in the mouth, water bottle, bath, or lotion. When taken in water, they can even be acceptable by lactose-intolerant people. There are homeopathic tissue salts in liquid-coated sucrose pellets for those who are lactose intolerant, if lactose cell salts used in water do not suffice. They are easily given to children, as most children like the sweet taste.

> *Cell Salts have enriched my practice. I recommend them for many acute and chronic ailments, and have seen my patients' health improve. The change is gradual, and I explain to my patients it may take several months. But, once they have experienced improvements, whereas over-the-counter or prescription drugs just cover up the problem, they return and ask how they work and are eager to continue their cell salts. These remedies are another medicinal tool I use to help people heal.*
> – Dr. Cindi Croft, D.O.

Some of the minerals in cell salts have many uses, including:
- **calcium** (3 forms) for bones, elastic tissue support, and digestion (assimilation)
- **iron** for oxygenating the blood, hemoglobin, and artery and vein strength

- **potassium** (3 forms) for nerve and brain function, mucus problems, and skin problems
- **magnesium** for all types of pain, especially neuralgia, and muscle spasms
- **sodium** (3 forms) for digestive power, body water balance, and high body-acidity
- and **silica** for bones, hair, skin, and connective tissue.

Most clients take the **tablets in a 12- to 24-ounce water bottle** that they sip all day. Each sip is a dose. The water chemistry creates a uniform mineral matrix that, when taken in this manner, allows you to overrule the usual homeopathic protocol to not drink with or following a dosage. However, cell salts are best when taken dry from the cap of the bottle to the mouth to avoid contamination (do not allow the cap to touch the lips). When using the dry method don't drink for 5 minutes before or after taking the pellets, and store them 3 feet away from electronic appliances to avoid electromagnetic fields rendering them useless. The many uses of cell salts follow this section (*See* Chapter 2).

Anyone can buy and use the 12 cell salts, separately or in combination, without fear of toxicity. This includes pregnant or nursing women; old or young alike; those taking medications; and even those using other natural therapies. Cell salts do not react with medications because they are supplying minerals on a cellular level.

Buy them individually or in a 12-bottle set to make formulas for your particular conditions. (*See* Chapter 5, Cell Salt Solutions, for combinations.)

Experience the power of cell salts for yourself, to get healthier; or use them as a tonic to improve your immune system. For more information, go to www.daveshealth.com.

> *I am certain that by adding cell salts to my daily routine, in addition to my normal vitamins and eating more raw foods, that I do have much more energy and I believe I feel a better mental balance and more harmony in my life.*
> – D. Michel, age 51

CHAPTER 2

The 12 Schuessler Cell Salts:
Your Comprehensive Guide

Learn about the benefits of each cell salt. In this section, you will find:

- Description of each cell salt: its purpose for the body.
- Location of the cell salt: where the cell salt is commonly found in the body.
- Function: the biochemistry of cellular health, as certain minerals create specific functions in the body.
- Common Uses: most frequent conditions that are benefited by the cell salt
- Modalities: the conditions that affect the body, based on time, temperature, emotions, etc. Watch for the symbol that tells what makes the condition become better (>) or worse (<).

Also included are descriptions about Bioplasma, and Biochemic Phosphates; two combinations I often recommend.

THE TWELVE CELL SALTS

#1 Calc Fluor (Calcium Fluoride)

Description: Calcium Fluoride is essential to the connective tissue of the body; for all conditions of tissue weakness, prolapse, or excessive hardness. It helps the tendons, ligaments, and joints of the body. Calc Fluor is used extensively for the teeth, instead of fluoride treatments for children, to strengthen enamel. Medical fluoride causes brittleness. Anywhere you find hardness of tissues, this remedy applies, which makes it valuable for cataracts of the eyes. Any extreme sagging of muscle or tissue also calls for this salt.

> *Calc Fluor helped to decrease all the facial signs of deficiency.*
> – B. Hansen, age 55

Location: Found in bone covering (Periosteum), teeth enamel, blood vessel walls, and skin cells.

Function: ELASTIC FIBER, formed by the union of calcium fluoride with protein and fats, it strengthens enamel – helps prevent tooth decay; gives elasticity/rebound to tissues, including the skin; also helps the body absorb hard lumps, especially on bone surfaces.

Common Uses: Bone problems; bone spurs; breast fibroids; cataracts; cysts; hemorrhoids; indigestion; cracking joints; weakness in lower back; enlarged lymph glands; deficient teeth enamel; varicose veins.

Modalities: Symptoms worse < cold, wet, change of weather, damp weather, sprains, beginning motion. Symptoms better > by continued motion, heat, applications of heat, rubbing.

#2 Calc Phos (Calcium Phosphate)

> *My nails started growing after a couple of years of splitting and breaking.* – J. Graves, age 31
>
> *Using Calc Phos along with "Teeth Roots" (Dave's homeopathic combination), people thought I had whitened my teeth.* – J. Felice, age 50

Description: Calcium Phosphate is used for bone health, injuries, and osteoporosis. Calcium metabolism, when disturbed, can cause osteoporosis or bone spurs (same problem, different manifestations). This salt treats both of them over the course of several months. It is also useful for teeth and digestive problems.

Location: Found in bones, cartilage, tendons, inner parts of teeth, and digestive fluid.

Function: BONE TISSUE. Calcium phosphate unites with protein and uses it as cement to build bone tissue. Bones are about 57 percent calcium phosphate. It also helps with assimilation problems, anemia, nerve pain, and more.

Common Uses: Anemia; arthritis; backache; bone inflammation; brittle or soft bones; broken bones; craving for smoked meats; diabetes; eczema; swollen glands; gout; headaches; hemorrhoids; hernia; incontinence; infections; swollen knees; lameness; nerves (pain): like electrical shocks; osteoporosis; smoking; cavities of teeth; teething problems; tonsillitis; toothache; worms.

Modalities: Symptoms worse < teething, loss of fluids, exposure to cold damp wind, thinking of symptoms, puberty, eating fruit, night. Symptoms better > summer warmth, dry weather, lying down, rest.

#3 Calc Sulph (Calcium Sulphate)

> *I had an impetigo blister that I would get on my chin. I took Calc Sulph and it cleared up.* – S. Price, age 37

Description: Calcium Sulphate is used for infections, pus, and general toxicity of the body. The discharges are yellow and filled with pus. This salt is used to detoxify the body and improve digestion (in my experience). Other uses are to finish, and clean up, chronic infections and improve the immune system.

Location: Found in skin (epithelial tissue) and in the blood (for clotting).

Function: SKIN & TISSUE SUPPORT. Calcium sulphate, by its union with protein, assists Kali Mur to form epithelial (skin) tissue, to hold it intact.

Common Uses: Acne; anal abscess; boils; burns; conjunctivitis; cradle cap; diarrhea; enlarged glands; hang nails; tendency toward infection; itching feet; mastitis; sore throat; yellow mucus discharges.

Modalities: Symptoms worse < dampness, drafts, stimulants, evening, sleep, menses. Symptoms better > open air, bathing, doubling over, uncovering.

#4 Ferrum Phos (Iron Phosphate)

Description: Ferrum Phosphate (iron) is important for oxygenation of the blood. It is very useful for low fevers and at the first signs of a cold or flu. It is the most useful for nose bleeds or other blood conditions, even hemorrhages. It is helpful for balancing iron in the body, whether it is high in some situations, or low in others, such as seen in pregnancy. It works to reduce anemia by helping the body to absorb iron.

Location: Found in blood (hemoglobin), vein and artery walls, and capillaries.

Function: OXYGEN CARRIER. The proper amount of Ferrum Phos in the blood carries oxygen to all parts of the body. Lack of oxygen increases circulation and creates excess heat.

Common Uses: Anemia; arthritis; bedwetting; bronchitis; cough; cystitis; diarrhea; earache; eye inflammation; low-grade fevers; head cold; headache; heart palpitations; hemorrhoids; hernia; hip inflammation; hoarseness; incontinence; indigestion; inflammations; injuries; morning sickness; stiff neck; nosebleeds; painful periods; pneumonia; prolapse; tinnitus.

Modalities: Symptoms worse < motion, noise, nights and 4 – 6 AM, suppressed perspiration, on right side of body, consuming sour foods, cold drinks, meat, and coffee. Symptoms better > cold, bleeding, lying down, rising, passing stools, and solitude.

> *Kali Mur and Mag Phos together helped with a recent bout of diarrhea.* – S. Snyder, age 53

#5 Kali Mur (Potassium Chloride)

Description: Potassium Chloride is used with medium fever conditions. It is useful for mucus conditions of the body, especially for mucus of the lungs with coughs, allergies, etc. The conditions for this cell salt are grey or thick white mucus.

Location: Found in blood-fibrin (protein).

Function: FIBRIN (fibrous protein). Kali Mur is the worker of the blood that forms fibrin and properly diffuses it through the tissues of the body. It keeps body fluids in correct thickness, including blood, and works on mucus conditions.

Common Uses: Acne rosacea; auto-immune diseases; blood clots; boils; bronchitis; bruising; canker sores; croup; cystitis; deafness; earaches; Eustachian tubes; facial redness; medium to high-grade fevers; chapped hands; head cold; heart palpitations; hip inflammation; indigestion from fats; kidney inflammation; morning sickness; mumps; nasal congestion; swelling; eczema; sore throat; white vaginal discharges .

Modalities: Symptoms worse < cold drinks, open air, drafts, night, dampness, sprains, motion, menses, fatty, rich foods. Symptoms better > rubbing, and letting hair down.

#6 Kali Phos (Potassium Phosphate)

> *I used Kali Phos for anxiety. I felt more aware of my stress levels. It helped keep them in check. I also pinpointed what made my anxiety levels too high and tried to deal with them in a different way.*– T. Thompson, age 29
>
> *I have had less stomach problems, i.e., bloating, stomach aches.* – S. Robbins, age 48
>
> *Kali Phos has made a big difference with me. Mentally I was less stressed. My thoughts were clear and I didn't feel so foggy.* – K. Couch, age 66

Description: Potassium Phosphate helps the nerves and gray matter of the brain. When the nerves are depleted by stress, we can experience sleeplessness or depression. Kali Phos is also used in pain and paralysis, fear, suspicion, weakness of memory. This remedy is for the anxious and nervous person. Nerves affected by Kali Phos are of the central nervous system.

Location: Found in the gray matter of the brain, and nerves.

Function: BRAIN. The basis of brain or nerve function is Kali Phos.

Common Uses: Anemia; asthma; brain injury; bad breath; canker sores; croup; cystitis; depression; dizziness; epilepsy; exhaustion; facial neuralgia; gangrene; nervous headaches; heart palpitations; hysteria; mastitis; light menstruation; dry mouth; nervousness; nosebleeds; sciatica; tinnitus; varicose veins; whooping cough.

Modalities: Symptoms worse < excitement, worry, fatigue, pain, cold dry air, mental or physical exertion, eating, early morning, puberty, being alone, sitting. Symptoms better > menses onset, sleep, eating, warmth, rest, gentle motion, cloudy weather, company.

#7 Kali Sulph (Potassium Sulphate)

> *Kali Sulph has helped in getting rid of ridges in my nails.*
> – C. Baker, age 44
>
> *Kali Sulph has caused a slight lightening of age spots.*
> – M. Baker, age 58

Description: Potassium Sulphate is specific to the third stage of inflammation or resolution. We find yellow discharges wherever there is a lack of sulphate in the system. There is breakdown of the skin and high fevers from infections or inflammations. This is the body's attempt to foster the bacteria to do their job of getting rid of self-inflicted toxins from a poor diet or polluted conditions of living in the modern world. When usage brings on sweating, it is near the end of the toxic condition. Kali Sulph is used for eczema, sinusitis, asthma, psoriasis, and more.

Location: Found in skin, scalp, and hair.

Function: OIL MAKER & DISTRIBUTOR. When this salt falls below the standard in quantity, oil and fats are improperly used and clog the pores of the skin.

Common Uses: Age spots; arthritis; brown spots; rattling mucus in chest; yellow dandruff; deafness; facial neuralgia; high-grade fevers; wandering pains; scarlet fever; vitiligo; yellow discharges.

Modalities: Symptoms worse < warm air, heated rooms, noise, evenings, consolation, after eating. Symptoms better > walking, cool air, fasting, open air, and heated room.

> *My cramps are considerably less during menstruation since taking Mag Phos.* – S. Krohn, age 45
>
> *Took sciatic pain away.* – J. Callahan, age 55
>
> *Mag Phos helped a lot with the redness in my skin. It took a lot of it away.* – M. Harvey, age 38

#8 Mag Phos (Magnesium Phosphate)

Description: Magnesium Phosphate is a nerve remedy also, but deals with muscular nerves and fibers. The symptoms are cramping, fast onset, primarily on the right side of the body. This mineral affects and feeds the heart and cardiovascular system. It is a great antispasmodic, useful for many areas of the body, including menstrual cramps. If symptoms are relieved by heat and pressure, this is a sign of the need for Mag Phos.

Location: Found in nerves (white fiber), muscles, and heart muscle.

Function: SPASMODIC CONDITIONS. The white fibers of nerves and muscles need Mag Phos to keep them in proper tune or function.

Common Uses: Angina; back chills; sharp pains in back; bed-wetting; bloating; child colic; colon cramps; darting pains; double vision; eczema; epilepsy; facial neuralgia; gas; neuralgic headaches; labor pains; leg cramps; menstrual cramps; neck pains; nightly aggravations; spasmodic cough; spasms.

Modalities: Symptoms worse < cold air, drafts, touch, nights, on right side, and from lying on right side, milk, motion, exhaustion. Symptoms better > heat, pressure, bending double, hot bathing, and friction.

#9 Nat Mur (Sodium Chloride)

> *Nat Mur seems to help with my headaches.*
> – P. Hamilton, age 41
>
> *Has helped with allergy symptoms of sneezing and runny nose.*
> – S. Wilcox, age 43
>
> *Nat Mur helped with my water retention and my shingle outbreaks while the Kali Phos helped with my stress levels.*
> – C. Tree, age 52

Description: Sodium Chloride, or common table salt, is one of the most famous cell salts for digestion, arthritis, and water distribution problems. The key is dryness of the mucus membranes or excessively watery discharges. Emotionally one sees grief and personal isolation. The person is very sensitive; prefers to be alone (for a defense). There may be malnutrition, constipation, anemia, and thin salty watery discharges from the body.

Location: Found in digestive system, blood (moisture), skin (moisture), kidney, and bladder.

Function: WATER DISTRIBUTOR. Water constitutes over 70 percent of the human body; therefore the carriers of water must be in like proportion.

Common Uses: Weak back and neck; bronchitis; canker sores; clear thin discharges; constipation; salt craving; deafness; depression; dryness; facial neuralgia; fear of emotions; fever blisters; grief; sweaty hands; hangnails; hay fever; throbbing headaches; heart palpitations; herpes I & II; introversion; parasites; sexual aversion; shy; greasy skin; loss of sense of smell; sneezing; loss of taste; teething with drooling; frequent urination.

Modalities: Symptoms worse < 9-11 AM, sun, heat, physical exertion, talking, writing, reading, bread, noise, music. Symptoms better > sweating, rest, open air, going without regular meals, and deep breathing.

#10 Nat Phos (Sodium Phosphate)

> *I noticed a difference [improvement] with gastrointestinal problems with Nat Phos.*– S. Krohn, age 45
>
> *I was amazed at how my ugly blemishes began to disappear using Nat Phos and Nat Sulph.* – J. Eggertson, age 58

Description: Sodium Phosphate governs the acid balance of the body. Alkalinity is health, and over-acid conditions allow for disease. The tongue often has a yellow mucus coating. Acid signs are seen as sour body-smell or sour-smelling discharges. Indigestion is a sign of lack of this salt. Candida infections, or vaginal yeast, as well as parasites come with over-acid conditions also.

Location: Found in stomach, mucus membranes, and lymphatic system.

Function: BODY ACID BALANCE. A certain amount of acid is necessary and always present in the blood. Excess acid is nearly always due to a deficiency of Nat Phos.

Common Uses: Acidity; acne; ankle itching; conjunctivitis; diabetes; hives; jaundice; morning sickness; parasites; pH imbalance; vomiting of sour fluids; yellow creamy discharges.

Modalities: Symptoms worse < milk, sugar, mental activity, during menses, thunderstorms, sex. Symptoms better > pressure, cold, and open air.

#11 Nat Sulph (Sodium Sulphate)

> *Nat Sulph and Kali Sulph have been shrinking a liver spot on my face.* – C. Baker, age 44
>
> *Nat Sulph helps with stomach aches.* – P. Hamilton, age 41

Description: Sodium Sulphate is responsible for liver health and is used for those with head injuries where one has become depressed and irritable. As with all sulphates, deficiency shows up as yellow discharges. This salt is responsible for helping the body to get rid of excess water. This is valuable for those with water retention. One can also use this for all kinds of hepatitis. Used for diabetes and also for asthma in children, especially in damp weather. This person may also be experiencing bad-smelling gas.

Location: Found in intercellular fluids.

Function: WATER REGULATOR. A deficiency of this salt prevents elimination of excess water in the tissues, blood and fluids, causing a water-logged condition.

Common Uses: Alcoholism; asthma; bloating; coughing; depression; diarrhea; gas; head injury; indigestion with bitter taste; liver problems; loose or huge stools; suicidal; sun sensitive; swelling; testicular swelling; excessive urination; vomiting of bitter matter.

Modalities: Symptoms worse < cold damp weather, head injuries, lying on the left side, light, music, vegetables, cold food and drink. Symptoms better > open air, passing gas, warmth, pressure, breakfast, sitting up.

#12 Silicea (Silica)

Description: Silica is responsible for connective tissue strength and the body's ability to rid itself of foreign objects. This is done by creating pus that discharges toxic waste. This remedy can dissolve scar tissue, and is very useful for keloid scars, skin problems, and vaccination reactions. Emotionally, those needing Silica are timid; their hands and feet are continuously cold. They often wear sweaters in the heat of the summer because of air conditioning.

I think that Silicea helped strengthen my back bones.
— D. Bytheway, age 73

Using Silicea, nails grew fast and long, moons started to show.
Skin seems to be smoother on face. — L. Miller, age 66

Ten years ago, I was in an accident and needed stitches in
my chin. Off and on over the years the scar has bothered
me. After taking Silicea for approximately three months,
my scar split and I removed two stitches. Using cell salts
can bring about amazing results. — J. Pettit, age 27

Location: Found in hair, skin, nails, periosteum (bone covering), nerve sheath, and bone.

Function: SURGEON. This salt is indicated in all suppurative (pus-forming) processes until the infiltrated parts have fully discharged the matter, to eliminate it from the system. It is also used for connective tissue support. Helps dissolve excess scar tissue.

Common Uses: Scarring from acne; boils; cold feeling; cysts; epilepsy; exhaustion; facial neuralgia; smelly feet; sweaty feet; head sweating; hemorrhoids; hip joint disease; infections; thin, breaking nails; sleepwalking; scars; shyness; timidity; ulcers; vaccination reactions.

Modalities: Symptoms worse < cold air, drafts, head uncovered, nervous excitement, new moon, milk, menses, night. Symptoms better > warmth, urination, and wrapping the head tightly.

TWO IMPORTANT CELL SALT COMBINATIONS

These cell salt combinations are commonly sold in health-food stores.

1. Biochemic Phosphates are the perfect combination to soothe the nerves. In this combination it contains Calc Phos, Ferrum Phos, Kali Phos, Mag Phos, and Nat Phos. Many people claim it helps with depression, anxiety, and panic attacks. It can be taken by itself or while using anti-depressant or anti-anxiety medications. There are no drug interactions as these are essential minerals in minute doses.

2. Bioplasma is a collection of all the cell salts conveniently packaged in one formula, used as a tonic to support and improve immune functioning. The body needs minerals for chemical and electrical health of the body. Most people use Bioplasma to support good health, detoxify, and rebuild mineral reserves. Use: Go slowly at first (by starting with only a few tablets) and increase little by little for maximum effect. Overuse can make the body detoxify too quickly.

> *I feel better overall since taking cell salts, but I have to say that the biggest difference I've noticed is that my face has cleared up a lot and I have less problems with breakouts and redness on my face, and that has improved my self-esteem and my emotional well being. – S. Krohn, age 45*

CHAPTER 3
Six Ways to Use Cell Salts
Inside and Out

Cell salts are versatile, and can be used in many different ways. These methods make it convenient for those with busy schedules. Use the method that works for you. See additional ideas for using cell salts externally on page 45.

FOR INTERNAL USAGE

1. Dry Method (in mouth)
Tap the right amount of cell salt tablets into the cap, and then drop the tablets into your mouth. They should **dissolve instantly** and taste good. Most people like the taste, even children. The most effective way to use cell salts is to take 2 to 20 tablets at a time, 1 to 3 times daily.

2. Wet Method (drinking)
There are almost no rules or precautions when using cell salts in any kind of water. Many people add their daily dose of cell salts (single type, or in a combination) into their water bottles, and sip a little all day long. The cell salts "energize" the water and create a true mineral water that won't clog up your veins or arteries, as some supplements do.

The bottle of water can be as small as a few ounces or as large as a gallon; size doesn't matter. Just finish the water within the course of the day; don't carry over for the next day. This method allows for higher water-intake and a smooth cell-salt delivery.

The better the water, the better the results, as pure water dissolves out toxins, improves the joints and your health in general. It is best to use **reverse osmosis or distilled water** as there are no hard minerals, again, to clog up the body. As one sips on the cell-salt water, every sip or swallow results in a substantial flow of assimilating minerals.

Drink your way to health and sooner or later it will show up on your face.

> *I believe everyone could benefit from the cell salts. It is hard to eat healthy – the cell salts help.* – S. Price, age 37

FOR EXTERNAL USAGE

3. Cell Salt Gels, Oils, Creams, and Lotions

Cell salts are versatile and can be used in various external ways. In Europe, cell salts are incorporated into creams and used on the skin. Remember, they work on a cellular level.
If you are a "do-it-yourself" kind of person, you can make your own gels or creams by taking your favorite cell salt or combination of salts, crushing the tablets into powder, and mixing the powder into a non-aromatic (fragrance-free) gel or cream.

Gels have the advantage of being water-based and non-sticky, and are easily absorbed into the skin. Aloe is a good one. In one ounce of your favorite gel, or lotion or cream, put 5 to 10 crushed cell-salt tablets and mix well. Then keep the container tightly closed. Some products absorb the salts better then others. Don't worry about the appearance of the paste you've made.

Oils don't absorb the cell salts very readily but are soothing to the skin. They can be used in fragrance-free massage oil.

Creams have the advantage of a slower delivery of cell salts to the skin. They have a time- release effect. The disadvantage is the sticky sensation that may happen. So, you may continue to rub them in for faster absorption.

Lotions as well as creams can be fragrance-free. Look for products that have simple ingredients and avoid those with chemical-sounding ingredients. Lotions tend to absorb quickly into the skin and can have the added benefit of moisturizing.

Use your cell salt gels, oils, creams, or lotions on **acupressure points, chakra centers, organ areas**, and **meridian lines as well as on sore or painful areas**. Just remember to consult a doctor if an area is very painful or sore for several days or weeks. Since cell salts are non-toxic, you can't make a mistake. Be adventurous and find the formulas that work best for you.

4. Cell Salt Poultice

Create a cell salt poultice: put 10 or more specific cell salts or a combination of salts (formula) in a quart of purified water, and stir or shake vigorously for 2 minutes. Put a soft cotton towel in this water and then wring out the excess. Put the cloth on the part of the body that you want to relieve. Use cold or warm water depending upon your need. You can put the cell salts into **cold water** for use on sunburns. (See the sunburn formula under the next section, Cell Salt Sprays.) **Hot water** poultices, with the right cell-salt formulas can soothe menstrual cramps, relieve pain, and more. You can also use the poultice over a particular organ or muscle.

5. Cell Salt Sprays

Put your cell salts into a spray bottle containing purified or distilled water. I would recommend using 10 tablets per quart. The advantage of spraying is that cell salts are absorbed directly through the skin, working at the cellular level. This is also good for those who are lactose intolerant. One of our customers likes to spray a wrinkle formula on her face before she goes to bed at night. For those with **anxiety** and panic, use Biochemic Phosphates (10 tablets per quart) to relax. Try this combination for **sunburn**: Calc Phos, Ferr Phos, and Kali Mur (3 tablets of each per quart).

> *I find several improvements in subtle areas—in little things that I had become so accustomed to feeling, I hardly notice anymore.* – S. Robbins, age 49

6. Cell Salt Baths

Enjoy the luxury and therapy of putting cell salts into your bath water. The cell salts disperse well into the water while the pores of the body open up to accept the minerals. Use 20 pellets of any cell salt in bath water, or use a combination that adds up to that number of tablets. For a general **detoxification bath**, put 20 tablets of the Bioplasma tablets into hot water. A simple strengthener for those with **osteoporosis** would be Calc Phos, Calc Fluor, and Silicea. You can put 20 of each, if you like.

A **pain formula** is Ferrum Phos, Mag Phos, and Nat Sulph.

A **relaxing bath** should have Mag Phos, Kali Phos, and Nat Mur.

To alleviate the discomfort of **menstrual cramps**, use Mag Phos, Kali Sulph, Kali Phos.

CHAPTER 4

Cell Salts for First Aid, Emergencies and Surgery

Cell salts are very useful in First Aid, emergency situations, and surgical preparations and healing. Use common sense in such situations, and alert a healthcare professional if you feel the need, and/or take the cell salts on your way to getting emergency treatment.

One of the easiest ways to use cell salts for emergency care is to put 10 tablets of each of the salts (those useful for that particular emergency) in a water bottle and sip every few minutes until pain or the condition improves. You may also use any of the other applications, internal or external, mentioned in this book.

Use your cell-salt kit of 12 remedies; mix and match for simplicity and ease of use. While cell salts are most commonly used in the 6x potencies, in emergencies any potency will work. Use 4 to 6 tablets every few minutes, or put 10 tablets of each into a quart of water and sip it all day. You can also soak a towel or soft cloth in a quart of cell-salt water and use as a compress over the injured parts.

These emergency remedies will not interfere with any medical drugs or treatments. All cell salts are non-toxic and will not interact or interfere with other herbs or medications. They can be used in children, adults, during pregnancy, and by nursing women.

COMMON EMERGENCIES	
Condition	**Cell Salt(s)**
Angina	Mag Phos, Kali Phos.
Bites and stings	Nat Mur, Nat Phos, Kali Phos; can use as a compress.
Bleeding	Ferr Phos, Kali Mur, Kali Phos.
Blisters	Nat Mur, Kali Phos, Ferr Phos; can use as a compress.
Bruises	Ferr Phos, Kali Mur; can use as a compress.
Burns	Ferr Phos, Kali Mur, Kali Sulph; can use as a compress.
Collapse	Kali Phos, Mag Phos, Nat Sulph.
Cramps	Mag Phos, Calc Phos.
Fractures	Calc Phos, Ferr Phos, Silicea (strengthens the bone; helps to avoid infections).
Head injury	Kali Phos, Ferr Phos, Nat Sulph.
Infections, acute	Kali Phos, Nat Phos.
Infections, chronic	Calc Phos, Calc Sulph.
Inflammation	Ferr Phos, Nat Phos.
Injuries	Ferr Phos (fevers), Kali Mur (prevent infections), Silicea (treat infections).
Knee Injuries	Calc Fluor, Ferr Phos, Nat Phos; can use as a compress.
Muscle strains	Kali Phos, Mag Phos.
Nerve Pains	Nat Mur, Mag Phos, Kali Phos.

Nosebleeds	Ferr Phos, Kali Phos, Nat Mur.
Shock and bleeding	Kali Phos, Ferr Phos, Calc Phos.
Spinal injuries	Mag Phos in hot water; sip as needed. May add Ferr Phos and Kali Phos.
Sprains	Ferr Phos, Kali Mur; can use as a compress.
Sunstroke	Nat Mur, Kali Phos, Kali Sulph.
Vomiting	Nat Phos, Nat Sulph, Ferr Phos.
Wounds	Ferr Phos, Kali Phos – every 2 hours.
Wounds-slow healing	Silicea, Calc Fluor.

Cell Salt Preparation: Pre-Surgery

Surgery is an injury, wound, and trauma to the body. Preparation starting weeks or months ahead is the best practice. Sometimes this is not practical. Check with your surgical healthcare professionals for possible problems with herbs and nutrients that may promote excess bleeding.

The cell salts, homeopathic remedies, and flower essences are safe in all circumstances and are to be used a few days in advance of surgery as well as afterward for a couple of weeks. Although your surgical team may not understand these, they are safe and you may need to make them aware. Make the following formula in an 8 – 32-ounce water bottle and sip all day, for maximum results. Use this formula for 14 days prior to surgery:

Pre-Surgery Preparation
- **Calc Sulph 6x – 3**
- **Ferr Phos 6x – 2**

- Kali Mur 6x – 1
- Kali Phos 6x – 5
- Mag Phos 6x – 7
- Nat Mur 6x – 5
- Silicea 6x – 2

Calc Sulph helps the body to detoxify.

Ferrum Phos is anti-inflammatory, oxygenating tissues for better healing.

Kali Mur is for secondary inflammation and to reduce mucus so the body can heal faster.

Kali Phos calms and heals the nerves. (Who wants to get cut anyway?)

Mag Phos relaxes the muscles and reduces cramping.

Nat Mur is for cellular integrity and anticipation stress.

Silicea helps prevent infections and deals with tissue integrity to prevent scarring.

Cell Salt Preparation: Post-Surgery

Based on your need, the following cell salts can be used individually or in combination for recovery from surgery. Or, simply continue to use the Pre-Surgery solution detailed above.

Calc Phos is for delayed healing especially with bone healing problems.

Calc Sulph is for excessive toxicity from anesthesia.

Ferr Phos is for a low fever and inflammation conditions.

Kali Mur is for respiratory, bronchial or excess mucus conditions.

Kali Phos is used for post-operative stress or nerve conditions.

Kali Sulph is for a stressed liver where there is irritability.

Mag Phos is used in muscle cramps or tightness.

Nat Mur is for depression, dryness or excessive watery-mucus conditions.

Nat Sulph is especially good for head surgeries and/or for depression after surgery. It supports the liver which is often a source of irritability.

Silicea is to prevent scarring and strengthen connective tissue. It helps to treat and prevent infection.

> *In the six months of participating in the cell salt study, the main thing that I have noticed is a general improvement in my feeling of well being. I wake up in the morning feeling more rested. I have a clearer mind, and more energy. The upper abdominal pain that shot through to my back has disappeared. I just have a better feeling, overall.*
>
> *– L. Arnold, age 53*

CHAPTER 5
Cell Salt Solutions: Combinations for Healing

Cell Salt Solutions are combinations of cell salts you can put together to satisfy the cellular needs of the body systems. Deficiencies in these systems cause symptoms, and then disease. Cell Salt Solutions provide the body with the necessary tools to heal.

It is best to use a combination of all the cell salts listed under each condition. You can use individual cell salts if indicated and add an extra one for specific conditions.

Stick with one Cell Salt Solution until the condition or disease improves. The results can show up in days, weeks, or even months for those with chronic conditions. Acute conditions usually respond within hours or days.

To make your Cell Salt Solution, put 10 tablets of each cell salt in a 12 – 24-ounce bottle of water and sip it all day. (Remember when starting out, you may use only a couple of tablets each and work up to 10 of each.)

> *The cell salts gave me more energy and helped me feel an overall better health. I also had more mental clarity when taking the cell salts. – C. Scavezze, age 27*

Abscess: a bacterial infection from poor immune function.
Calc Sulph – clearing infection

Ferr Phos – inflammation
Kali Mur – swelling
Silicea – chronic infections

Acne, teenage: May come from poor eating habits and hormonal issues.
Calc Sulph – detoxification and infection
Ferr Phos – inflammation
Kali Mur – white mucus discharges
Nat Mur – clear discharges

Anemia: A complicated issue that causes a low iron condition. Iron supplements often constipate because of iron toxicity.
Calc Phos – stimulates bone marrow for red blood cell
    production
Ferr Phos – iron absorption
Nat Mur – iron absorption

Anxiety caused by stress and nervous condition. Females should explore hormone issues.
Kali Phos – in all nervous conditions
Mag Phos – muscular tension
Nat Mur – anxiety from grief

Appendicitis: An inflammation of the appendix. The appendix protects the large intestine from colon cancer. Put solution in hot water and sip every few minutes. May also put a compress containing solution directly over the appendix area.
Ferr Phos – inflammation, low fever
Kali Mur – inflammation, medium fever
Mag Phos – antispasmodic

Arthritis: Painful inflammation of the joints.
Nat Phos – acidity in the body
Ferr Phos – inflammation, and fevers
Kali Mur – to dissolve mucus
Silicea – to dissolve scar tissue, and stop infections

Asthma: Chest tightness and inability to breathe.
Kali Phos – stress induced
Nat Sulph – damp weather
Mag Phos – chest tightness or spasms
Kali Sulph – worse from heat

Back Pain: Lower back.
Calc Phos – bone support
Ferr Phos – inflammation
Nat Phos – muscular strains due to over-acid conditions
Silicea – connective tissue

Bad Breath: Comes from bad digestion.
Nat Phos – digestion, acidity
Nat Sulph – liver support, digestion
Kali Phos – digestion associated with stress

Bed Wetting: Inability to hold the urine at night.
Calc Phos – to increase nerve strength of the bladder
Ferr Phos – inflammatory conditions
Kali Phos – nervous conditions
Silicea – shyness or infection

Blood Pressure: For high blood pressure continue medication, and slowly come off drugs under a doctor's supervision, while using the cell salt solution.

High Blood Pressure: Caused by a stressful lifestyle.
Calc Fluor – connective tissues
Ferr Phos – inflammation, and fevers
Silicea – connective tissue
Kali Phos – nervous high blood pressure

Low Blood Pressure: Caused by nervous conditions.
Biochemic Phosphates – Supports the nerves and strengthens the cardiovascular system.

Boils: Toxicity that comes to the surface of the skin. May use as a pack to promote suppuration.
Calc Fluor – hard boils
Calc Sulph – pus, yellow discharges
Silicea – pus discharges

Breasts: Inflammation, lumps, fibroids.
Calc Fluor – hardness
Calc Sulph – toxicity
Ferr Phos – inflammation
Kali Mur – congestion
Silicea – connective tissue

Candida Albicans: A genus of yeast (fungi family). Its function is to control carbohydrate metabolism. Given enough unrefined sugars, it will take over and create a multitude of symptoms which are too numerous to explain here. Discharges are seen on the tongue, or are vaginal.
Nat Phos – acidity, creamy discharges
Calc Sulph – toxicity, yellow discharges
Nat Sulph – liver support, yellow discharges

Carpel Tunnel Syndrome: Inflammation of the tendons of the wrists.
Calc Fluor – connective tissue
Calc Phos – tendon support
Ferr Phos – inflammation
Mag Phos – muscular pain

Cataracts: Calcium deposits on the eyes. Use as long as the eyes don't get worse. It may take several months.
Calc Fluor – proper calcium absorption
Calc Sulph – toxicity
Nat Phos – over-acidity
Silicea – calcium deposits, scars

Cavities: Prevention is best, but this may help minor cavities. Use for several months in water, sipping all day.
Calc Fluor – enamel integrity
Calc Phos – bone integrity
Silicea – bone integrity, infection

Chicken Pox: A childhood disease designed to mature and strengthen the immune system. The cell salts help the immune system to clear the body faster.
Calc Sulph – toxicity, yellow discharge
Ferr Phos – inflammation, first stage
Kali Mur – inflammation, second stage, mucus conditions
Nat Mur – watery discharges

Cell salts seem to cleanse my system. They have a detox effect. I feel more balanced and stabilized.

— C. Koch, age 41

Colds: Usually from bacterial condition, from toxicity. The bacteria have the job to carry away the toxins. These cell salts help the body to reduce toxins.
Ferr Phos – inflammation, low fever
Kali Mur – mucus congestion, medium fever
Nat Mur – clear runny discharges
Add Calc Sulph, only if discharges are yellow

Colic: Indigestion in babies, but also helpful in adult digestion. Put in water and give a few drops on the tongue every few minutes; reduce the frequency as symptoms improve.
Nat Sulph – bad gas
Kali Sulph – liver, digestive support
Mag Phos – to relax the bowels

Constipation: Normally, you should have 1 to 3 bowel movements a day. If not, use more fiber; flax or psyllium fiber is desirable.
Kali Mur – to remove mucus
Nat Mur – excessive dryness
Nat Phos – to remove acidity
Nat Sulph – to support the liver

Cough: Respiratory weakness caused by various reasons.
See also **Lungs.**
Ferr Phos – anti-inflammatory
Kali Mur – lung support, mucus dissolving
Kali Sulph – liver involvement

Cramps (muscular) and female cramping during menstruation. Use in hot water for fastest results.
Calc Phos – digestive cramps

Kali Phos – nervous cramps
Mag Phos – muscular cramps

Cystitis: Bladder inflammation with urgency, stinging and burning.
Nat Phos – over-acidity
Ferr Phos – inflammation
Kali Mur – mucus and inflammation
Mag Phos – spasms, muscles

Deafness: Hearing loss from various reasons.
Calc Sulph – from infections, mucus, toxicity
Ferr Phos – inflammatory reasons
Kali Mur – mucus congestion
Silicea – scar and connective tissue
Kali Phos – nerve deafness

Depression: Prolonged sadness; this combination may be used along with any medication and counseling.
Kali Phos – nervous and depression conditions
Nat Mur – sadness and grief
Nat Sulph – sadness, suicidal feelings

> *I now believe in cell salts and their benefits to maintaining a healthy body whereas before the study I thought that it was all a hoax.* – B. Hansen, age 55

Diabetes: Blood sugar stays too high. Adult-onset diabetes.
Ferr Phos – inflammation, stress on the pancreas
Nat Phos – blood sugar, over-acidity
Nat Sulph – liver, pancreas support

Diarrhea, caused by various reasons (could be liver or stomach problems).
Ferr Phos – inflammation
Mag Phos – spasm pain
Nat Sulph – liver support

Earaches: Middle ear congestion and pain. Safe for everyone.
Ferr Phos – inflammation
Kali Mur – Eustachian tube blockage
Mag Phos – sharp ear pains

Exhaustion, mostly from stress. This combination helps pick up the energy.
Biochemic Phosphates – nervous exhaustion
Add Nat Mur – for grief situations

Fevers, especially in children: Use as long as you feel safe without other professional medical help; or take the person to a doctor. Cell salts can be used along with doctor's medications. Add Calc Sulph for detoxifying. Use these cell salts individually or together as a combination.
Ferr Phos – low fevers (102°F or lower)
Kali Mur – medium fevers (102°F - 104°F)
Kali Sulph – high fevers (103°F - 106°F)

Fingernails: Breaking, thin, brittle, crumbling.
Calc Fluor – brittle or thin and brittle
Calc Phos – thin
Silicea – thin or thick, brittle, crumbling

Gallstones: A hot pack (cloth, soaked in cell-salt solution) placed on the gallbladder area overnight, may also be useful.

Kali Sulph – liver/gallbladder support
Nat Phos – digestion, over-acidity
Nat Sulph – liver/gallbladder support
Silicea – connective tissue integrity

Gas: Flatulence from indigestion, or liver, or gallbladder problems.

Calc Phos – to promote digestion
Kali Mur – to get rid of mucus
Mag Phos – cramps (gas)
Nat Sulph – liver support, bad smelling gas

Hair Loss: Alopecia is hair loss in spots. There are many reasons for hair loss; often it is hormonal.

Kali Phos – nerves
Nat Mur – dryness, or watery discharges
Silicea – brittle hair, baldness

Hay fever: Allergic conditions. Discontinue dairy products.

Calc Sulph – detoxification, yellow discharges
Ferr Phos – inflammation
Kali Phos – nervous conditions
Nat Mur – watery discharges

Cell salts have helped to heal my seizures and increase my energy and sense of well being. – S. Hollingshead, age 46

Heart tonic: to strengthen the heart. Will not interfere with prescription medications.
Kali Phos – nervous conditions
Mag Phos – strengthens heart muscle
Nat Mur – emotional heartache

Hemorrhoids: Painful burning and anal itching, usually due to a weakness in the blood vessels of the anal region, and blood and liver toxicity.
Calc Fluor – connective tissue
Ferrum Phos – inflammation
Silicea – connective tissue

Hips: For pain, and hip joint disease.
Calc Phos – bone and nerve health
Ferr Phos – inflammation
Kali Mur – congestion
Mag Phos – muscular health
Silicea – bone, connective tissue

Hot Flashes: Menopausal symptoms of heat and flushing.
Ferr Phos – low-grade inflammation and heat
Kali Phos – nervous conditions
Kali Sulph – hormonal issues and sweating
Silicea – inflammations associated with hot flashes and heat in general

Hypoglycemia: Pancreatic weakness, low blood sugar. Shakiness when hungry.
Calc Phos – digestive help
Kali Phos – nervous conditions
Nat Phos – over-acidity, digestive conditions
Nat Sulph – liver and pancreas support

Incontinence: Urine leakage, often in women when laughing or coughing, etc.
Calc Phos – tissue and nerve integrity
Kali Phos – nervous conditions
Kali Sulph – liver and hormonal components

Indigestion, caused by poor diet choice or lack of sufficient stomach acid.
Calc Phos – digestive support, to normalize stomach acid
Kali Phos – nervous indigestion
Nat Mur – digestive support
Nat Sulph – liver support, gas

Indigestion with a bitter taste in mouth (gallbladder involvement).
Nat Sulph – gallbladder support
Calc Sulph – detoxification
Kali Sulph – gallbladder support

Indigestion: Nervous stomach.
Nat Phos – over-acidity
Calc Phos – digestion, normalizes stomach acid
Kali Phos – nervousness

Kidneys: For weakness, excessive urination.
Calc Phos – nerve support
Ferr Phos – inflammation
Nat Phos – over-acidity
Kali Sulph – inflammation

Liver Problems, often characterized by anger and irritability.
Kali Mur – congestion
Kali Sulph – liver support
Nat Sulph – liver and digestive support
Silicea – connective tissue support

Lungs: For coughs and congestion. *See also* **Coughs. Lung problems are often a sign of grief or sadness.**
Calc Phos – nervousness
Ferr Phos – inflammation
Kali Mur – lung mucus and congestion
Silicea – connective tissue, inflammations and infections

Menopause: Symptoms of weight gain, bloating, tiredness, lowered sex drive, etc.
Calc Phos – digestion support
Kali Phos – nervous conditions
Kali Sulph – hormonal issues

> *As a woman after menopause, I am grateful for cell salts. I was not happy with the choices I had from my medical doctor. Cell salts have made it possible for my body to regulate and feel good; also I can lead a happy mentally stable life.*
> – J. Thelin, age 54

Menses, heavy bleeding.
Calc Phos – blood builder
Ferr Phos – iron, and inflammation
Kali Phos – nerve support
Kali Sulph – hormone, liver support
Nat Mur – blood builder

Menses, painful. Avoid a heavy meat and dairy diet.
Ferr Phos – inflammation
Kali Phos – nerve support
Mag Phos – cramping pains

Morning Sickness: Nausea during pregnancy. Safe at all times.
Kali Phos – nervousness
Nat Mur – digestion
Nat Phos – over-acid conditions

Muscle Pains: May also be used externally in a gel or cream.
Ferr Phos – inflammation
Mag Phos – muscular pain or cramping
Nat Phos – over-acidity
Silicea – connective tissue integrity

Nasal Congestion: This formula helps the body to remove mucus. Stay away from dairy products and sweets.
Ferr Phos – to reduce nasal inflammation
Kali Mur – to reduce mucus and congestion
Nat Mur – to reduce dryness with congestion

Nausea: Generalized indigestion.
Ferr Phos – inflammation
Kali Phos – nervous stomach
Kali Sulph – liver disturbances
Nat Sulph – liver toxicity or weakness

Pain: General pain formula.
Ferr Phos – inflammation

Mag Phos – sharp shooting pains, cramping
Nat Sulph – liver support
Silicea – infectious condition, splinter-like pains

Parasites and worms. This formula reduces toxicity so the parasites don't have a job.
Calc Phos – nerve conditions
Calc Sulph – toxicity
Mag Phos – nerve conditions
Nat Phos – over-acidity (worms feed on mucus and acidic conditions)

> *Using the cell salts, I noticed as my body was more balanced that my mind was more clear, which allowed me to be more emotionally balanced.*
> – B. Skovensky, age 34

Self esteem, low.
Kali Phos – nervous conditions and depression
Nat Mur – grieving and depression
Silicea – timidity

Thyroid problems: Basedow's disease.
Ferr Phos – inflammation
Kali Phos – nervous conditions
Mag Phos – muscle and heart conditions
Nat Mur – metabolism and thyroid

Toothache pain, for various reasons. In acute conditions, put in hot water and sip as needed.
Calc Phos – calcium absorption

Ferr Phos – inflammation
Mag Phos – sharp pains

Weight loss: Use in conjunction with food reduction and daily exercise.
Calc Phos – digestion, proper stomach acid production
Nat Mur – emotional eating
Kali Phos – nervous eating
Nat Phos – toxicity, acidity

CHAPTER 6
Cell Salt External Uses

The **cell salt creams** can be used in acute cases every hour or so, and in chronic conditions, 3-4 times a day. These need to be used for several days to several months for most effective cell salt absorption and symptom alleviation. If used overnight, a thick paste can be applied, covered by plastic and a towel or cloth, as not to soil the sheet.

In wet eczema or open wounds, the **crushed tablets can be applied.** Try this on small areas first. Use the tablets straight on the wet eczema, or add a small amount of water to form a paste.

Hot compresses made with cell salt water often give relief to pain and fever. For fevers, use a towel soaked in hot water: use 20 cell salt tablets in a pint of water. The towel is put on the calves of the leg to reduce the fever. This pack is then covered with a large dry towel. This method can be used with the appropriate cell salt or combination for most painful parts of the body. Afterward, you can put on the cell salt cream.

For burns, sunburns, insect bites, bronchitis, and liver problems: I recommend putting 10 to 20 pulverized tablets of the recommended cell salt into 3-6 ounces of plain yogurt; spread the mixture on the affected part, at least ½-inch thick, and then cover with plastic.

> *I was amazed at my overall health improvement, my energy level raised.* – J. Lassig, age 31

CELL SALT EXTERNAL USES	
Ailments in alphabetical order	
Abdomen, pressure of the upper abdomen	Nat Sulph
Abscesses	Calc Sulph, Kali Sulph, Silicea
Acne	Nat Phos
Acne Rosacea	Kali Mur
Acne, infected	Silicea
Age spots or brown spots	Kali Sulph
Anal eczema with severe itching	Nat Mur
Arthritic complaints	Nat Sulph
Arthritis (weather change type)	Calc Phos
Bells palsy (facial paralysis)	Kali Phos
Blackheads	Nat Phos
Bleeding	Kali Mur
Boils	Calc Sulph, Silicea
Bone infections	Silicea
Bone wounds	Calc Sulph
Bones, broken	Calc Fluor, Calc Phos
Respiratory weakness	Calc Phos
Bruising	Ferr Phos, Kali Mur
Burns, first degree	Calc Phos, Ferr Phos

Burns, second degree	Kali Sulph
Choking	Mag Phos
Colic cramps (apply to stomach)	Mag Phos
Colon disturbances with stomach pain	Nat Sulph
Connective tissue inflammation	Kali Mur
Connective tissue weakness	Calc Fluor, Calc Phos, Silicea
Cough	Calc Sulph
Cramps	Mag Phos
Cramps with bloating	Mag Phos
Diseases with infections and pus	Silicea
Ear infections (apply behind ear)	Silicea
Eczema	Calc Phos, Kali Mur
Eczema with blisters and severe itching	Nat Mur
Eczema, wet in spots	Nat Sulph
Elastic tissue weakness	Calc Fluor
Eustachian tube blockage (apply behind ear and down neck)	Kali Mur
Eyelid twitches	Mag Phos

Eyelids, hanging skin under lower eyelids	Nat Phos
Fatty large pores	Nat Phos
Feet, burning (neuropathy)	Calc Sulph
Feet, numbness of	Nat Mur
Frostbite	Nat Sulph
Gallbladder, cramping	Mag Phos
Glands, swollen	Kali Mur
Gout	Nat Phos
Growth pains in children (legs)	Calc Phos
Growths, abnormal	Calc Fluor
Hair loss, circular	Kali Phos
Hands, numbness of	Nat Mur
Hangnails, infected	Kali Sulph
Hardening of tissues	Calc Fluor
Headache	Silicea
Headache from mental effort (apply to forehead)	Calc Phos
Headache that starts at the neck, with sticking pains	Mag Phos
Heart cramps	Mag Phos
Heart disturbances	Nat Sulph

Heart pains (stitching)	Kali Phos
Heart palpitations	Ferr Phos, Nat Mur
Heart palpitations from over exhaustion	Kali Phos
Heartburn upon least movement (rub on upper stomach)	Ferr Phos
Heartburn with bitter taste (apply over stomach)	Nat Sulph
Hemorrhoids	Calc Fluor
Hip pain	Mag Phos, Silicea
Infections	Kali Phos, Silicea
Inflammation	Ferr Phos
Inflammation, advanced	Kali Mur
Inflammatory conditions, chronic	Kali Sulph
Injuries	Ferr Phos, Kali Mur
Insect bites	Nat Mur
Joint pains	Calc Phos
Joint spasms	Mag Phos
Joints and fingers, cracks of	Nat Mur, Silicea
Joints, cartilage destruction	Calc Fluor
Kidney inflammation	Calc Sulph
Knee inflammation	Kali Mur

Leg eczema on lower legs	Nat Mur
Leg sores, lower leg (especially in the elderly)	Kali Sulph
Leg ulcers	Silicea
Leg wounds, gangrene	Kali Phos
Ligaments damaged	Silicea
Lips cracked	Nat Mur
Liver disturbances	Kali Sulph
Liver problems	Nat Sulph
Liver spots	Kali Sulph
Menstrual cramps	Mag Phos
Migraines (apply to temples or painful parts)	Mag Phos
Mouth, cracked corners of	Nat Mur
Muscle inflammation	Kali Mur
Muscle pains	Ferr Phos, Mag Phos
Muscle weakness	Kali Phos
Nasal mucus congestion (apply over sinuses)	Kali Mur
Neck aches	Silicea
Neck, weak	Nat Mur
Nerve pains	Kali Phos, Mag Phos
Neuralgia	Mag Phos
Pain	Ferr Phos, Mag Phos
Pores, large	Nat Mur, Nat Phos

Pus	Silicea
Rectal fissures	Calc Fluor
Rectal muscle	Kali Phos
Restless legs	Ferr Phos, Kali Phos
Rheumatism	Nat Phos
Rib inflammation	Kali Mur
Scarring	Calc Fluor, Silicea
Scoliosis	Calc Fluor
Shaking of joints and muscle groups	Mag Phos
Sinus inflammation	Calc Sulph
Sinus problems	Kali Mur
Skin chafed	Nat Mur
Skin cracks	Calc Fluor, Silicea
Skin hanging under lower eyelids	Nat Sulph
Skin, dry withered	Nat Mur
Skin, lack of pigmentation (vitiligo)	Kali Sulph
Skin, thin sagging	Silicea
Spasms of joints and muscle groups	Mag Phos
Spinal disc damage	Silicea
Spinal discs bulging	Calc Fluor
Sprains	Kali Mur

Stomach cramps	Mag Phos
Sweating	Nat Mur, Silicea
Tendonitis	Kali Mur
Throat, choking	Mag Phos
Varicose veins	Calc Fluor, Kali Mur
Vein inflammations	Kali Mur
Wounds	Kali Mur
Wounds, infected	Kali Sulph
Wrinkles, facial	Silicea

EXTERNAL USES FOR EACH CELL SALT

CALC FLUOR is used for connective tissue disturbances, weakness, or hardening.
External Uses:
>   Broken bones
>   Cracks of the skin
>   Elastic tissue weakness
>   Growths, abnormal
>   Hardening of tissues
>   Hemorrhoids
>   Joints, cartilage destruction
>   Rectal fissures
>   Scarring
>   Scoliosis
>   Spinal disc problems
>   Varicose veins

CALC PHOS concerns the protein metabolism of the body. Works for bone health, tendons, cartilage, skin, mucus membranes, blood, and the brain.
External Uses:
    Arthritis (weather change type)
    Bones, broken
    Bronchioles, weak
    Burns, first degree
    Connective tissue weakness
    Eczema
    Growth pains in children (legs)
    Headache from mental effort (apply to forehead)
    Joint pains

CALC SULPH is for infective processes and pus conditions. This salt works to thin the blood, and get rid of excess acidity; helps wound healing.
External Uses:
    Abscess
    Kidney inflammation
    Boils
    Bone wounds
    Cough
    Feet burning (neuropathy)
    Sinus inflammation

FERR PHOS, iron, works on the muscle cells of the tissues and heart as well as stomach and colon wall musculature. It builds the blood. Builds the hemoglobin and normalizes acidity of the cells. It supports the immune system, and detoxifies.

External Uses:
    Bruising
    Burns, first degree
    Heart palpitations
    Heartburn upon least movement (rub on upper stomach)
    Inflammation and pain
    Muscle pains
    Restless legs

> *Cell salts helped with my jittery leg problem – helped me to fall asleep easier.* – S. Wilcox, age 43

KALI MUR has to do with the thickness of bodily fluids (blood also). It works on the skin and serous membranes. It affects the mucus membranes, tendons, and joint cartilage, as well as rib inflammation.
External Uses:
    Acne rosacea
    Advanced inflammation
    Bruising, sprains, bleeding
    Connective tissue inflammation
    Eczema
    Eustachian tube blockage (apply behind ear and down neck)
    Glands, swollen
    Injuries
    Knee inflammation
    Nasal mucus congestion (apply over sinuses)
    Muscle inflammation
    Rib inflammation

Sinus problems
Tendonitis
Vein inflammations and varicose veins
Wounds

KALI PHOS is one of the most important cell salts. It strengthens the ability of the cells to divide. Good nerve remedy. Strengthens the heart muscle and calms down the nerves. It is a universal remedy.
External Uses:
Bells palsy
Circular hair loss
Heart pains (stitching)
Heart palpitations from over exhaustion
Infections
Leg wounds, gangrene
Muscle weakness
Nerve pains
Rectal muscle

KALI SULPH is a detox remedy. It supports the detoxification organs such as the liver, kidneys, skin, and mucus membranes. This is an anti-inflammatory of the highest order. We see the thick, yellow, slimy secretion. Other signs of need for this cell salt include discharges of a cold from the ears, nose, and sinuses and infected tissue; infected conditions of the skin and secondary connective tissue.
External Uses:
Abscesses
Age spots or brown spots
Burns, second degree
Chronic inflammatory conditions

Infected hangnails
Infected wounds
Liver disturbances
Lower leg sores (especially in the elderly)
Skin, lack of pigmentation (vitiligo)

MAG PHOS is a nerve remedy. This is often used in conjunction with the other phosphorus remedies. Magnesium is needed to bind carbon dioxide. Magnesium is needed for correct electrical function of the nerves.
External Uses:

Colic cramps (apply to stomach)
Cramping of the gallbladder
Cramping pains of the nerves
Cramps
Cramps with bloating
Eyelid twitches
Headaches that start at the neck, with sticking pains
Heart cramps
Hip pains
Menstrual cramps
Migraines (apply to temples or painful parts)
Neuralgia
Shaking and spasms of joints and muscle groups
Stomach cramps
Throat choking

NATRUM MUR controls water in the body. This controls swelling or dryness of the body. The deficiency shows up in the skin and mucus membranes. The typical signs are burning in the stomach, dry tongue, dry throat, larynx, clear thin mucus, great thirst, scratchy throat, and dry cough.

External Uses:
- Anal eczema with severe itching
- Chafed skin
- Cracked corners of the mouth
- Cracked lips
- Cracking joints
- Dry withered skin
- Eczema with blisters and severe itching
- Insect bites
- Lower leg eczema
- Numbness of hands and feet
- Pores, large
- Sweating

NATRUM PHOS helps the body get rid of toxins through the urinary tract. This release of protein toxins is through uric acid, sugars in milk sugar, and fats through fatty acids. These signs are seen in the skin, mucus membranes, as well as muscle and lymph tissues.

External Uses:
- Acne
- Blackheads
- Enlarged greasy pores
- Gout and rheumatism

NATRUM SULPH sends the water of the tissues to the kidneys and also metabolizes byproducts. Symptoms include pressure of the liver and gastrointestinal disturbances, often combined with stomach pain and a bitter taste in the mouth.

External Uses:
- Arthritic complaints

Colon disturbances with stomach pain
Frostbite
Hanging skin under lower eyelids
Heart disturbances
Heartburn with bitter taste (apply over stomach)
Liver problems
Pressure of the upper abdomen
Wet eczema in spots

SILICEA is a connective tissue remedy, working on the connective tissue cells directly, also on the collagen and elastic tissues. It works to prevent and treat wrinkles, and to prevent signs of old age. Silicea is used for weakness of the immune system. Used for weak and anxious children. It has a direct effect on the white blood cells. It has an effect on the absorption of cellular byproducts, diseases and foreign substances. It works on infections, pus, and scar tissue, and helps build white blood cells.
External Uses:

Abscess
Boils
Bone infections
Damaged ligaments
Diseases with infections and pus
Ear infections
Facial wrinkles, thin sagging skin
Hip pain
Infected acne
Leg ulcers
Neck and headaches
Spinal disc damage
Sweating

CHAPTER 7
Facial Signs of Cell Salt Deficiencies

Facial diagnosis for cell salt deficiencies was pioneered by Dr. Schuessler (1821-1898) and was verified and expanded by Dr. Hickethier (1891-1958). Various practitioners in Germany, such as doctors, homeopaths, and pharmacists, have done further work in this area. Very little has been written on this topic in English. I have started to disseminate this material in English and hope the English-speaking world will catch on to this simple way to detect cell salt deficiencies. In my other books on cell salts (see www.hohmpress.com), you will find color pictures and in-depth descriptions of each of the cell salts with their guiding symptoms showing deficiencies in the body.

Facial diagnosis is a method of observing cell salt deficiencies by specific appearances in the face. Deficiencies are revealed, in particular, by:

- Color: excess color (red, yellow, brown), or a lack of pigmentation.
- Lines: their location, direction, and depth.
- Texture: raised features, appearance, bloating, pores (large), or dandruff.
- Shine: polished, gelatinous, or high-gloss.

> *Thanks for the opportunity to participate in this study. I probably wouldn't have been as faithful doing this on my own. Improvements I have noticed are: smoothness of skin, fingernail ridges are more smooth, forehead lines not as deep, and I sleep better.*
>
> – C. Visser, age 62

CALC FLUOR facial signs include blue lips, brownish-black circles under the eyes, white skin flakes, and translucent tips of teeth; raised or fan-shaped wrinkles around the eyes, as well as cracked lips.

CALC PHOS facial signs are a yellowish waxy appearance, translucent tips of teeth, and white flakes in the teeth or fingernails. There is also a stretched-skin appearance on the cheekbones, and small or thin lips.

CALC SULPH facial signs are an alabaster or dirty-white coloring along the lower face or jaw line. There can also be liver spots or brown spots on the face.

FERR PHOS facial signs are seen as bluish-black circles under the eyes. Acutely, we see red cheeks and ears, in fever conditions. One also sees a sleepless or hung-over appearance. Chronic iron conditions are seen in anemia, which can show as paleness in the face.

KALI MUR facial signs shown in the face are a milky appearance to the skin; this may be mixed with red, purple or blue. I have seen much success in using Kali Mur with acne rosacea with underlying spider veins, as well as raised bumps just below the shoulders on the upper arms.

KALI PHOS facial signs show in an ashen-gray appearance as well as a dull appearance of the eyes (they don't sparkle). One also can see, in more chronic conditions, sunken temples or cheeks. Bad breath and body odor (nervous sweat) is also a sign.

> *The little things on my face, it seemed to help them fade or blend in. My whole body health has improved!*
> — J. Peay, age 65

KALI SULPH facial signs are seen as brownish-yellow pigmentation of the nose-mouth area. Liver spots, pregnancy mask, freckles, or a lack of pigmentation (vitiligo).

MAG PHOS facial signs are seen as blushing, in acute conditions. In chronic situations we see a constant redness of the cheeks of a bright "magnesium redness" of a longstanding character on the nose; this can especially be seen in those with liver damage, including alcoholics.

NAT MUR facial signs are seen in a gelatinous appearance in the lower eyelid border. The hair line is often red and greasy. Large pores are a sign of deficiency of this salt, as well as dandruff, puffy cheeks and a bloated appearance.

NAT PHOS facial signs are seen in blackheads and a greasy combination skin. Yellow raised pimple-like bumps around the eyes. The chin is red. Cheeks have dry or greasy appearance.

Rings or metal jewelry can cause discoloration on the skin because of over-acidity.

NAT SULPH facial signs include a slight greenish cast in acute conditions, as well as a yellow eye sclera. There are signs of swollen lower-eye bags. In chronic conditions, where the liver is damaged, a swollen purplish-red nose will appear, again, especially in alcoholics.

SILICEA facial signs include a glossy polished shine, as a bald man has, and wrinkles of the skin. Silica deficiency has specific wrinkles that run parallel to the ears, crows feet, and more. Generally, you will see deep-set eyes. Hair may be brittle, along with fingernails and toenails. This deficiency is also seen as red eyes.

> *I feel more energetic. I think my skin has brightened up and cleared up some.* – M. Frantz, age 38

CHAPTER 8

Cell Salts for Detoxification Using the Seasons of the Zodiac

Dr. George Carey first introduced the concept of cell salts allied with the Zodiac signs. His concept encompassed taking a cell salt associated with the Zodiac sign of your birth, as your body would probably use up more of that cell salt than the others (thus becoming deficient in it); and further, to use the cell salt to cleanse the body during that Zodiac-sign's time of year (or its season).

To use either of these ideas, put 10 tablets in a bottle or cup of water and take sips all day. The following is a list of each salt, seasons of the Zodiac and the areas of the body they work on:

Season	Zodiac	Cell Salt	Areas of Detoxification
January 20 to February 18	Aquarius	Nat Mur	Legs
February 19 to March 20	Pisces	Ferr Phos	Feet, Lymphatics
March 21 to April 19	Aries	Kali Phos	Head
April 20 to May 20	Taurus	Nat Sulph	Neck
May 21 to June 20	Gemini	Kali Mur	Arms, Nervous system

June 21 to July 22	Cancer	Calc Fluor	Breast, Stomach, Spleen
July 23 to August 22	Leo	Mag Phos	Heart, Lungs, Liver
August 23 to September 22	Virgo	Kali Sulph	Intestines
September 23 to October 22	Libra	Nat Phos	Stomach, Kidneys
October 23 to November 21	Scorpio	Calc Sulph	Sex organs, Urinary organs
November 22 to December 21	Sagittarius	Silicea	Thighs, Hips, Buttocks
December 22 to January 19	Capricorn	Calc Phos	Knees, Spleen, Skin

I was skeptical about the difference that taking cell salts would actually have on my life. I realize now, that they have made a difference. I feel that my body has performed more efficiently. I also noticed that there has been less illness in my life.– D. Scavezze, **age 31**

CHAPTER 9
Additional Testimonials

In response to the questions: "How has this cell salt challenge affected your health?" or, "How has taking cell salts affected your health?" participants said:

Didn't get sick all winter! – J. Magner, age 52

I think it made me feel more energetic and mentally balanced. All my white spots in fingernails went away. – D. Michel, age 51

Had no allergies this season, for the first time in years.
— R. Miller, age 67

I was really happy when my face started clearing up and it's not so red any more. It has more of a healthy-looking color to it.
— A. Osgothorpe, age 20

If you can treat an ailment and see improvement, it helps in your self-esteem, and I believe this is what helped me.
— K. Oshiro, age 44

I have gone off all prescription drugs and I am doing great.
— E. Pierce, age 67

Less puffiness under my eyes. – M. Revill, age 72

I just seem to have more energy. – C. Scavezze, age 27

I feel healthier and have a better vision of life. The cell salts have helped my immune system and my digestion.
— D. Scavezze, age 31

I have appreciated the opportunity to learn a new way to be proactive in taking care of my health. – B. Skovensky, age 34

When I remember to take them I sleep better and feel more energetic and mentally alert. – S. Wilcox, age 43

I feel calmer and more peaceful in traffic. The pain in my upper abdomen [unidentified source] has almost completely stopped. Liver spots and moles are fading – some are almost gone. More energy, clearer thinking. Happier. – L. Arnold, age 53

I have felt a lot better. My skin has not been as dry.
— K. Bowen, age 61

My hair, nails and skin are also much better.
— J. Callahan, age 55

It has helped me remain alert and the feelings of stress, although I have had more challenges this way, have remained more stable or recovery has been rapid. – K. Couch, age 66

My skin seemed to improve. Age spots lightened and lines decreased.
— M. Cox, age 54

Overall better health. – J. Felice, age 50

I feel more energetic. I think my skin has brightened up and cleared up some. – M. Frantz, age 38

It's made me more aware of my body/symptoms. I have a better understanding of minerals and their effect on our bodies. Cell salts have helped to regulate my system better. I'm grateful for this option. – J. Graves, age 31

While on the cell salts I felt more in control of the stress and fatalistic feelings that seemed to plague me. I also saw my face begin to take on a healthier look. – B. Hansen, age 55

It made me more regimented and has affected my spiritual life.
– D. Healy, age 53

Stabilized my moods, lessened my perspiration, skin tags clearing up. – C. Koch, age 41

Energy increased, better attitude, digestion – less acidity. – S. Koch, age 50

My face cleared up a lot and that has improved my emotional state. I seem more able to do sports with less problems than I've had in the past. – S. Krohn, age 45

BIBLIOGRAPHY

Anshutz, E.P., *A Guide to the Twelve Tissue Remedies of Biochemistry*. New Delhi, India: B. Jain Publishers (P.) Ltd., reprint edition 2003.

Card, David R., *Facial Diagnosis of Cell Salt Deficiencies*. Prescott, Arizona: Hohm Press, 2005.

Chapman, Esther, *How to Use the Twelve Tissue Salts*. Martius Lane, London, England: Thorsons Publishers Limited, re-printed 1968.

Phatak, S.R., *Repertory of the Biochemic Remedies*. New Delhi, India: B. Jain Publishers (P.) Ltd., reprint edition 2003.

Powell, Eric F.W., *Biochemic Prescriber*. Rustington, Sussex, England: Health Science Press, 1960.

Powell, Eric F.W., *Biochemistry Up to Date*. Morden Surrey, England: The Albion Press, 1963.

Schuessler, W.H., *The New Biochemic Handbook*. Saffron Hill, London, England: New Era Laboratories LTD, reprint 1970.

INDEX

ABOUT THE AUTHOR

David R. Card is a certified nutritionist with a bachelor's degree in psychology from the University of Utah. He is a certified homeopath from the Hahnemann Academy of North America, under the direction of Dr. Robin Murphy, N.D., and has a master herbalist certificate from the School of Natural Healing.

David is a native of Alberta, Canada, and has been involved in the health and nutrition industry since 1980. He resides in Salt Lake City, Utah, and is the author of two books, *Facial Diagnosis of Cell Salt Deficiencies* (cell salts/minerals) and *Seven Symbols of Healing* (planetary astrology).

His focus is to educate, giving the community the ability to take charge of their health and have greater vitality. David continues to research and study, sharing information in his classes and seminars.

CONTACT INFORMATION

Dave's Health & Nutrition
1817 W. 9000 S., West Jordan, Utah 84088
(801) 446-0499
www.daveshealth.com
info@daveshealth.com